History of
HOSPITAL POINT

Pioneer Medical Center
1899-1920
Province of Bocas del Toro, Panama

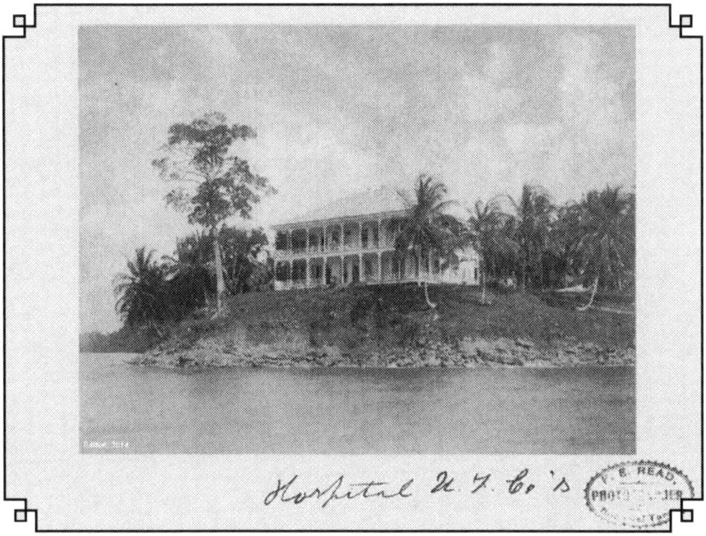

History of
HOSPITAL POINT

Pioneer Medical Center
1899-1920
Province of Bocas del Toro, Panama

Clyde S. Stephens

Cecropia Press

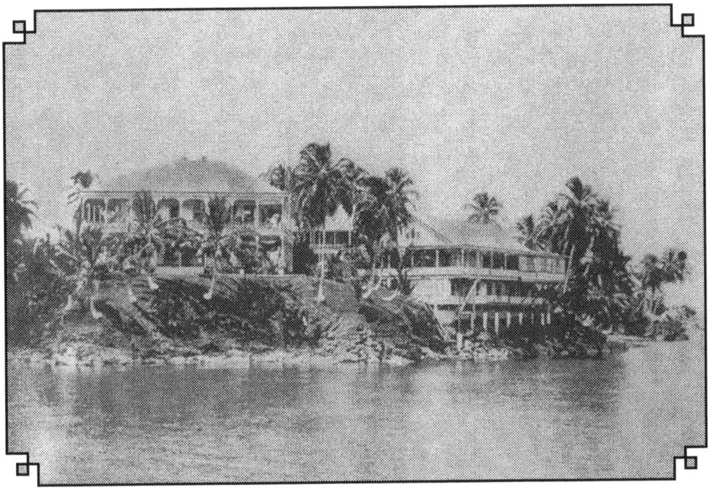

Hospital Point, Bocas del Toro, Panama
Circa 1914

New edition, Cecropia Press, 2023
Edited by Patricia Alvarado
Title page photograph by F. E. Read, New Hospital, 1900.

362.11
St43 Stephens, Clyde S.
The history of Hospital Point : Pioneer Medical Center, 1899-1920, Province of Bocas Del Toro, Panama / Clyde S. Stephens. -- Panamá : Cecropia Press, 2023.
90 p. ; 20 cm

ISBN 978-9962-715-40-5

1. HOSPITAL POINT (BOCAS DEL TORO)
2. HOSPITALS – PANAMÁ – HISTORY
I. Title.

ISBN: 9789962715405, soft cover, English
ISBN: 9789962715412, ebook, English
ISBN: 9789962715429, soft cover, Spanish
ISBN: 9789962715436, ebook, Spanish

Cecropia Press
cecropiapress.com

Dedicated to my parents,
Carl Wilson Stephens and Era Mae Bullock Stephens,
who planted the seed of curiosity
and taught me the pleasure of learning.

History of Hospital Point

CONTENTS

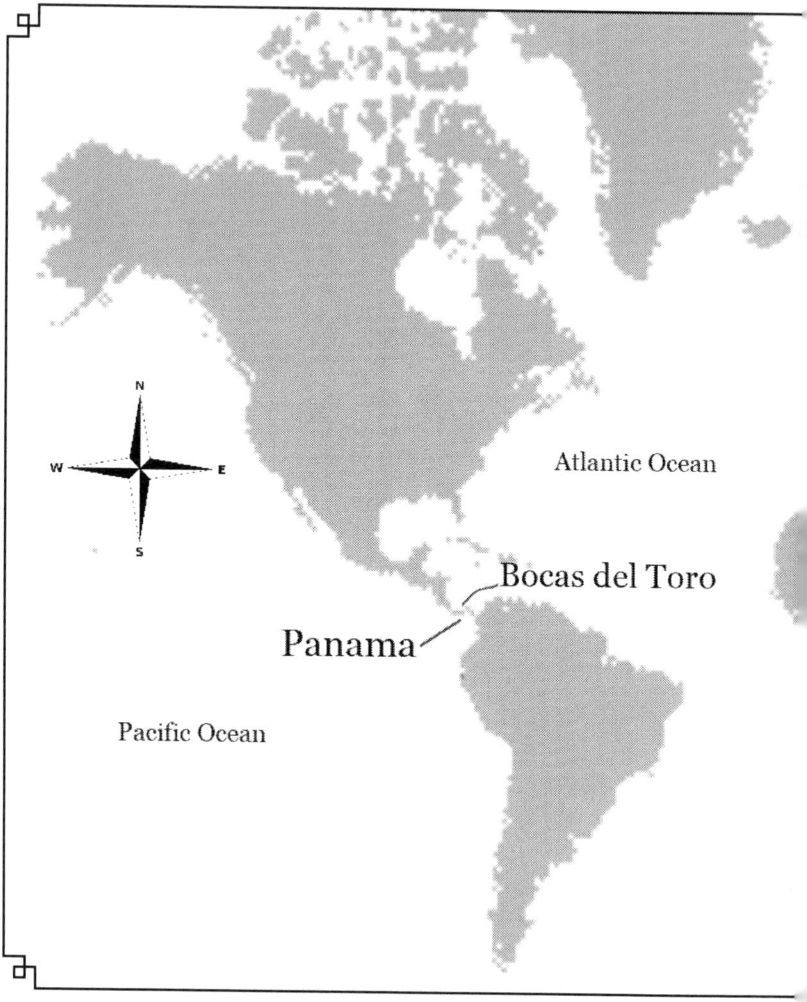
N
W
E
S
Atlantic Ocean
Bocas del Toro
Panama
Pacific Ocean

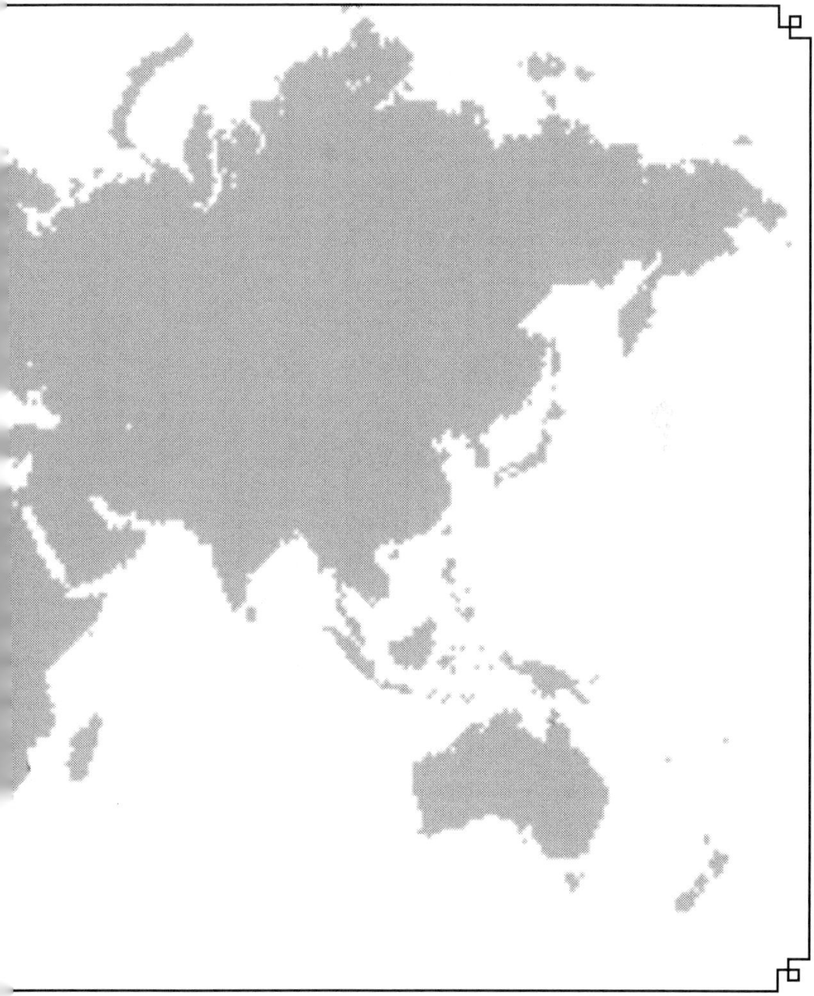

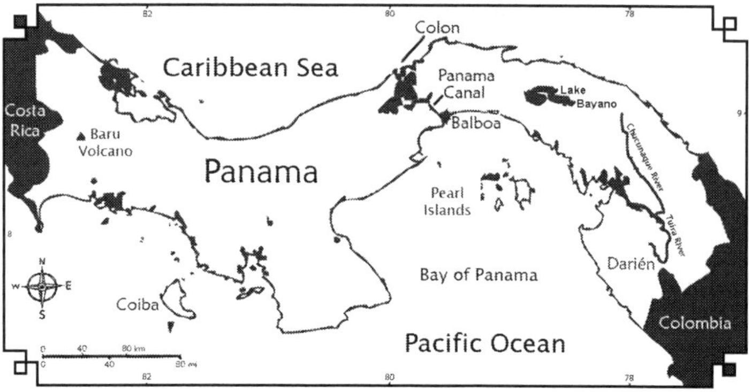
82
80
78
Colon
Caribbean Sea
Panama
Canal
Lake
Bayano
Costa
Rica
Baru
Volcano
Balboa
Panama
Pearl
Islands
Chucunaque River
Tuira River
N
W
E
S
Darién
Bay of Panama
Coiba
Colombia
Pacific Ocean
0 40 80 km
0 40 80 mi

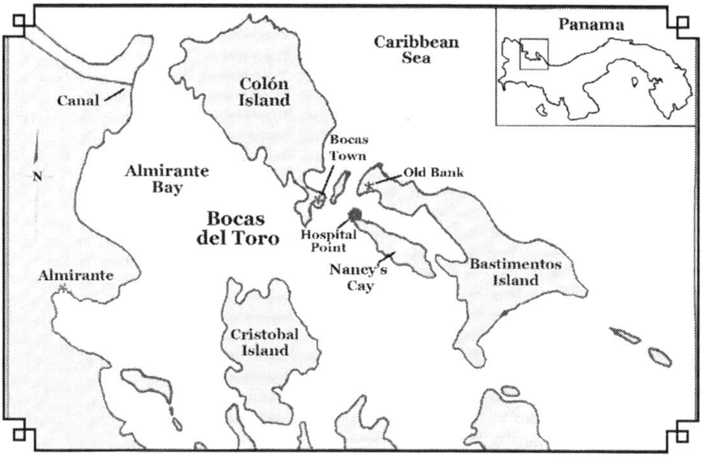
Panama
Caribbean
Sea
Colón
Island
Canal
N
Almirante
Bay
Bocas
Town
Old Bank
Bocas
del Toro
Hospital
Point
Nancy's
Cay
Bastimentos
Island
Almirante
Cristobal
Island

Introduction

HOSPITAL POINT IS ON the western tip of Nancy's Cay in the archipelago of Bocas del Toro, Panama, at latitude 9º 20' North and longitude 82º 13' West. Christopher Columbus sailed by the island during his fourth voyage in 1502,[1] but, contrary to local beliefs, references have not been found to prove that the explorer named the islands and waterways in the archipelago.[2,3,4] As English-speaking buccaneers, pirates, traders and settlers appeared during the next three centuries, the island became known as Nancy's Cay. During his excursions in 1817, Orlando Roberts wrote about Nancy's Cove and Provision Island (*Isla Bastimentos*) where he visited turtle fishermen from Corn Island and San Andrés Island.[5] In the medical records of the United Fruit Company dated 1899-1920, the island is referred to as Nances Cay.[6] At some point in time, this name may have been derived from *nances*, a common fruit tree on the island. In Spanish, the island is known as Solarte, but it is not known when this name was given.

Pre-Columbian artifacts found by the author in 1993-95 on the north shore of Nancy's Cay at Pine Creek, 250 meters from the point, were estimated by archaeologist Carlos Fitzgerald to be approximately 1,000 years old. Indigenous people inhabited much of this area when Columbus sailed through the archipelago, but populations declined because of tribal wars and European diseases.[7] Since the Spaniards never gained control of the region, a few English-speaking people from the Caribbean began to settle on the islands in the early 1800s.[8] American planters initiated the first banana plantations on the islands and along the rivers.[9] By the end of the century, the banana business surged and immigrants of many nationalities arrived to benefit from the prosperity of this new industry.[10] With them came numerous sanitation and health problems.[11]

Several banana companies operated in Bocas del Toro during the late nineteenth century. Some of these were: Jochen Ludwig Heinrich Hein, Snyder Brothers Banana Company, Camors, McConnell and Company, and Minor C. Keith. Banana communities developed along the Chiriqui Lagoon at Cricamola, Chiriqui Grande, Robalo, Pumpkin River, and Monkey Cay, but the largest center of commercial operations was at the city of Bocas del Toro on Columbus Island (*Isla Colón*). Here, the narrow strip of beach filled up fast with businesses and houses. As thousands of newcomers arrived, the town expanded over the pestilent mudflats and mangrove swamps behind the shoreline, thus creating a severe public health crisis.

Fortunately, in 1881, the Cuban doctor Carlos Finlay made the historic discovery that mosquitos transmitted yellow fever. However, it was two decades later before his finding was recognized. In 1897, in India, malaria was found in mosquitos by Ronald Ross. Soon after, medical authorities accepted the fact that mosquitos were vectors of yellow fever and malaria. By isolating victims and destroying mosquito breeding habitats, these devastating diseases could be controlled if money and technology were made available. Consequently, that was what the United Fruit Company did.

Before this time, no major efforts had been made to control deadly tropical diseases along the Caribbean coast. During the French endeavor to construct the Panama Canal from 1882 to the end of the century, despite good French doctors and hospitals, about 25% of the canal labor force died from malaria, yellow fever and other tropical scourges, which was one of the major reasons for the French canal failure.[12] This and other examples made the United Fruit Company recognize that its investments were at great risk unless public health was successfully managed.

By 1899, the giant United Fruit Company of Boston superseded all other banana interests in the region and established its headquarters in the city of Bocas del Toro. To enable the company to expand and do business, a medical department was established to assure a healthy and functioning labor force. As a result, the western tip of Nancy's Cay was chosen as the site for a medical center which became known as Hospital Point.

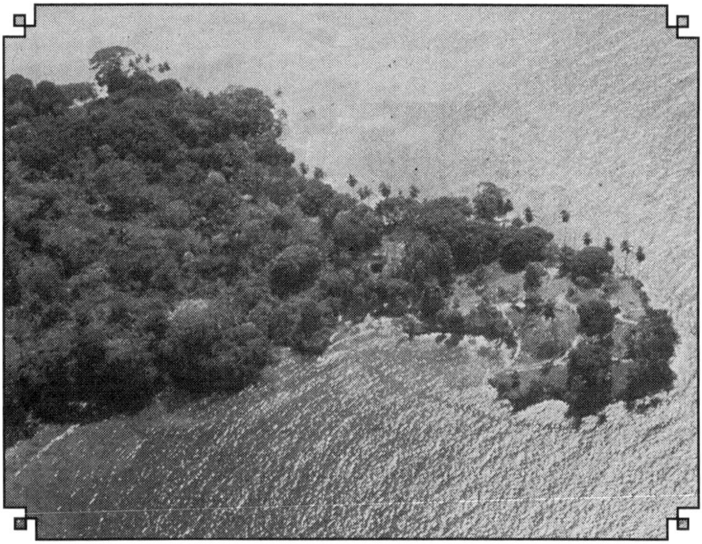

Hospital Point, 1971

Nancy's Cay

THIS FORESTED ISLAND IS seven kilometers long and runs approximately east and west. Climatically, the region has no pronounced dry season, although there is less rainfall in September/October and February/March. Rains peak in July and December. Average annual precipitation is 2,515 mm and mean temperature is 28° C. Hospital Point is surrounded by coral reefs which drop into deep channels. Waves from the open Caribbean break on the reefs and the cliff at the point. Prevailing winds cool Hospital Point and reduce the nuisance of mosquitos and sand flies, thus creating a healthier environment. The island is two kilometers east of the city of Bocas del Toro which isolated the medical center from a major source of disease and health problems. Before development by the United Fruit Company, Nancy's Cay was sparsely populated by a few Creole families near the point.

Early Records and Medical Facilities

THE FOLLOWING IS QUOTED from the first medical director, Dr. Robert Earl Swigart, in his United Fruit Company Medical Department review covering 1899-1911:

> The Hospital service of the United Fruit Company of Bocas del Toro was installed August 20, 1899, with a resident surgeon at Chiriqui Sanitarium, Monkey Cay, Chiriqui Lagoon, on whose shores were the properties of the various planters which were taken in as a part of the United Fruit Company. There were employed 2,020 men, and the sanitary conditions at Rio Caucho, Robalo, Chiriquicito, and Cricamola were very bad. Little was known then of proper sanitary methods, and malaria and yellow fever were rampant. The first two years proved the worst in the history of the Company, with a death-rate of

over 5 percent per annum among white people treated. As there were no hospital accommodations for colored people, a record to their death-rate was impossible. The new building at Nances Cay, the present site of the hospital, was erected June 23, 1900. To accommodate the development of Chiriquicito, Cricamola, and Robalo, branch hospitals were maintained at these places for a period of two years. The branch hospital at Chiriquicito accommodated 60 colored patients, that at Robalo, 35; and the one at Cricamola, 20. These hospitals were closed only when the project was abandoned, and efforts were concentrated in Changuinola. In this new district, a hospital was opened for colored people, accommodating 70 laborers, and was maintained for nearly four years. Up to the month of September, 1904, services were rendered to the negroes as out-patients, and it was not until after this date that we opened our hospitals to this class of labor. The service in Changuinola has been replaced with sick-camps and dispensaries, and at present there are seven of this type to supply laborers with first aid, the one central hospital providing treatment for those who are not promptly relieved through Dispensaries and Sick-camps.[13]

The Medical Center at Hospital Point

IN 1900, THE UNITED Fruit Company rebuilt a hospital previously constructed on Nancy's Cay by Minor C. Keith, an American businessman, railroad, banana plantation and shipping magnate in Costa Rica, Colombia and Panama.[14] Captions on early photographs of the hospital referred to the facility as Quarantine Island.[15] Soon after construction, Colombian Conservative forces took over the hospital in 1901 and 1902 and used the point as a headquarters and assault base against the Liberals on the neighboring island of Bastimentos during the War of a Thousand Days.[16]

When Panama gained independence from Colombia on November 3, 1903, officials of the new government of Panama were invited by the United Fruit Company to visit Bocas del Toro, which included a trip to the hospital. The excursion took place on March 24-29, 1904. Members of the party included Tomas Arias, F. V. de la Espriella, Julio J. Fabrega, Manuel Quintero, Luis de Roux, F. Mutis Duran, Federico Boyd and son Archibaldo Boyd, and a newspaper reporter from *La Estrella de Panamá*. They were joined in the Bocas del Toro capital by Governor Juan Jose Diaz. The assitant manager and local German merchant, Herbert Leer, and the company manager, John Morgan Kyes, represented the United Fruit Company. Doctor Robert Earl Swigart received the group at Nancy's Cay and gave a tour of the hospital.[17]

The facility was described in *La Estrella de Panamá* newspaper as having a main hospital with an annex. The main hospital normally accommodated six administrative patients. It was also the residence of Dr. Swigart, and included a kitchen and a pharmacy. Sick laborers were treated in the annex where the reporter noted 63 patients during the tour.

At the same time, on March 28, 1904, Minor C. Keith, vice president of the United Fruit Company, came from Limon, Costa Rica, with his engineer, M. H. Peyroutet, for a meeting with the new government delegation. They agreed that United Fruit Company engineers and government engineer Harmodio Arosemena would draw up a formal, revised plan for the pestilent city of Bocas del Toro. The plan called for a sewer system, streets and a park. A concrete wall would be built around the city in order to retain a land fill which would be pumped from the bottom of the bay. This would greatly improve sanitation and public health in the new provincial capital and banana boom town, only two kilometers across the pass between Hospital Point and Careening Cay.

Sometime after 1904, the Colored Hospital was built for the labor force. Also, a huge home was built on the west slope of the point for the division manager, and later, for the doctors. These and other buildings, sidewalks, a passenger dock and a cargo dock are shown in photographs taken in 1910. In 1914, a new building for surgery, a laboratory, a pharmacy and an office were constructed.

When the medical center was fully developed, there were 16 buildings crowded onto the narrow, rugged point which measured only 0.8 hectare, as shown on a property map copied in 1911 from the original. This uneven terrain peaks at nine meters above sea level and is composed of heavy clay mixed with limestone gravel and coral rock strata.

Hospital Point became a showcase that attracted numerous visitors. Many photographs and descriptions appeared in reports and books of the day. In 1969, the author restored old photograph albums found in the United Fruit Company archives in Almirante and made negatives of photographs of the medical center. These original albums disappeared a few years later.

During the first decade of the twentieth century, banana plantations on the islands and shorelines died from a fungus wilt called Panama disease and the business shifted to the alluvial floodplains of Changuinola, Sixaola and the Talamanca Valley. Before the Changuinola River railroad bridge was finished in 1908, the sick and dying had to travel by rail to a boat on the Changuinola River, transit the Snyder Canal to Bocas del Drago, then cross Almirante Bay to Hospital Point. This made Hospital Point a remote and difficult destination for patients, especially those that had to travel 125 kilometers from the Talamanca Valley in Costa Rica. Consequently, a more convenient hospital was built on the mainland at the banana port of Almirante where patients came directly by rail from the plantations. Architectural plans for the Almirante hospital were shown in the 1919 *Annual Report* and the new medical facility was opened in September, 1920.[18] At this time, the entire medical center on Nancy's Cay was closed after only two decades of use. Buildings were razed and soon the jungle covered the island point for half a century.

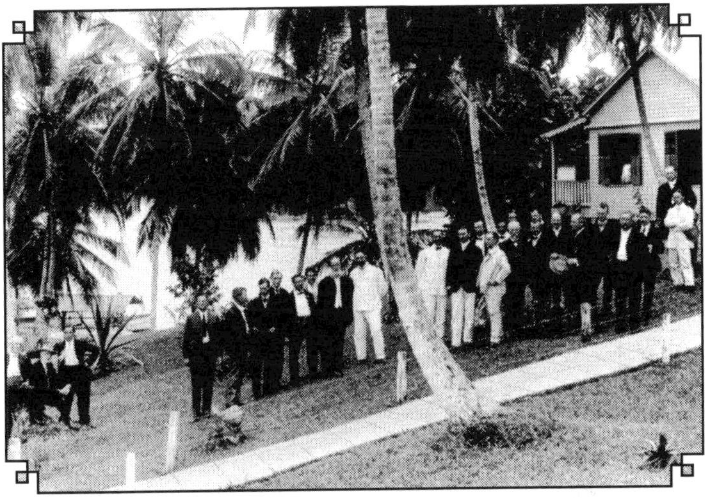

Above: Medical doctors from Mobile and New Orleans visiting Hospital Point in 1906 assessing yellow fever control in Bocas del Toro.

Below: Medical doctors and staff in 1906 hosting visiting doctors at Hospital Point.

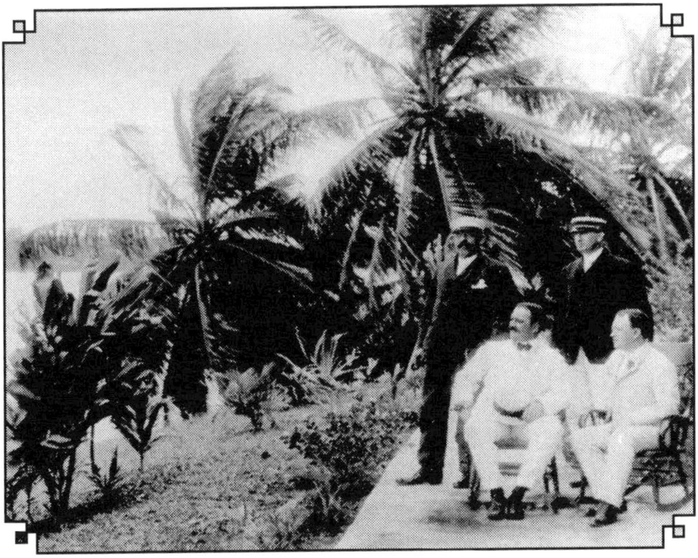

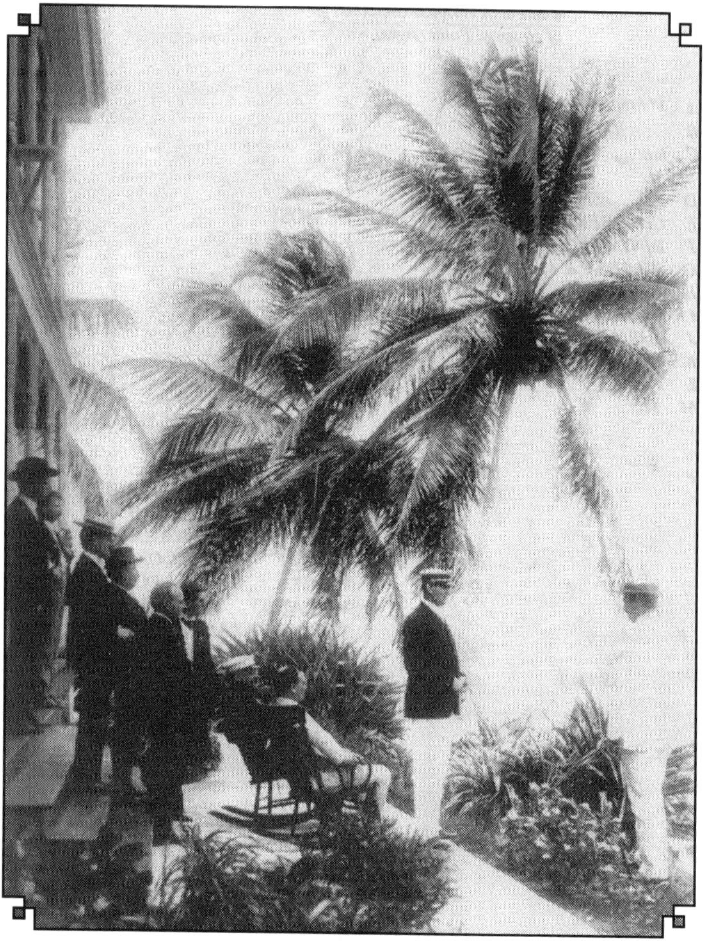

Medical doctors and United Fruit Company officials hosting public health team in 1906 on the north side of the hospital.

Description of the Buildings

IN 1993, A SURVEY and map of Hospital Point were made to show the location of each original building, concrete sidewalks, steps, docks and other facilities. The drawing of each building site was based on the presence of numerous concrete foundations. Each building is identified by a capital letter on the map and is referred to in the text.

Main Hospital

This building was 7.7 meters above sea level and was on the tip of the point facing north with a view of the Caribbean. It became a landmark and was a favorite subject for photographers. The hospital was for administrative employees, mostly Americans and Europeans. There were living quarters on the first floor for doctors and nurses.

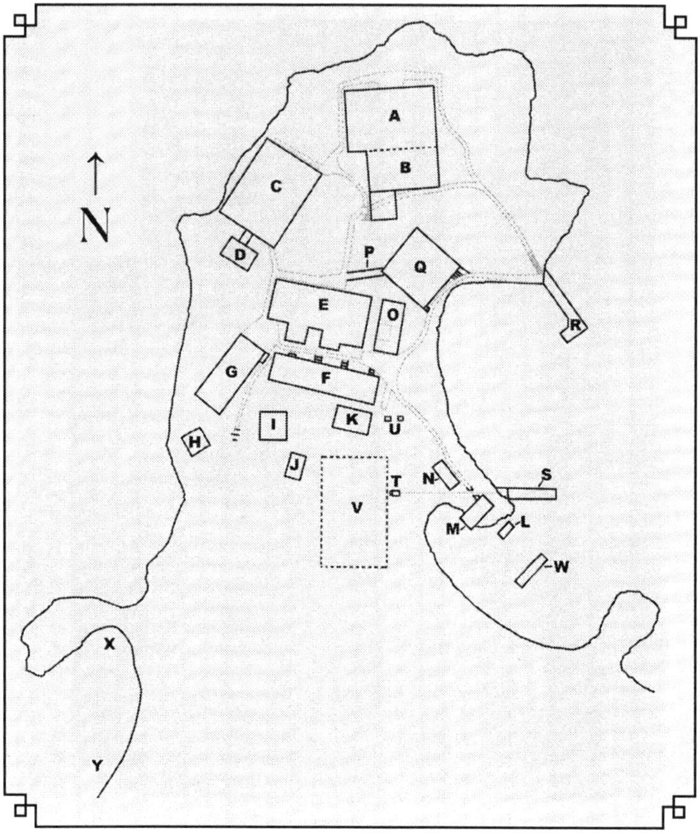

Map of Hospital Point

A. Main Hospital, B. Annex,
C. Residence of Manager/Medical Superintendent, D. Kitchen,
E. Colored Hospital, F. Dining Room/Kitchen, G. Wards 3 & 4,
H. Cottage, I. Laundry, J. Dormitory, K. Workshop, L. Toilet,
M. Morgue, N. Carbide Gas House, O. Warehouse/Ice House,
P. Covered Sidewalk, Q. New Surgery Building,
R. Passenger Dock, S. Cargo Dock, T. Winch for Coal Car,
U. Electric Generator, V. Tennis Court, W. Dead Skiff,
X. Peyne's Chinese Store, Y. James Tong's Store.

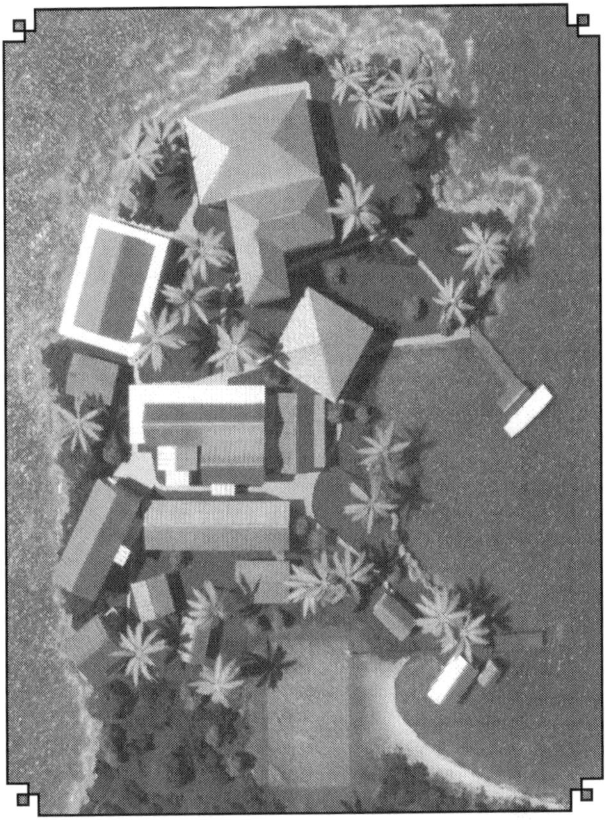

Hospital Point showing full development before 1920.

Annex

This large building, attached to the south side of the Main Hospital, was built over a steep slope and depression. A single-story room on the east side was the Sanitary Office. A laboratory and pharmacy occupied the first floor until these facilities were moved south across the sidewalk to the new surgery building in 1914. The upper floor was a hos-

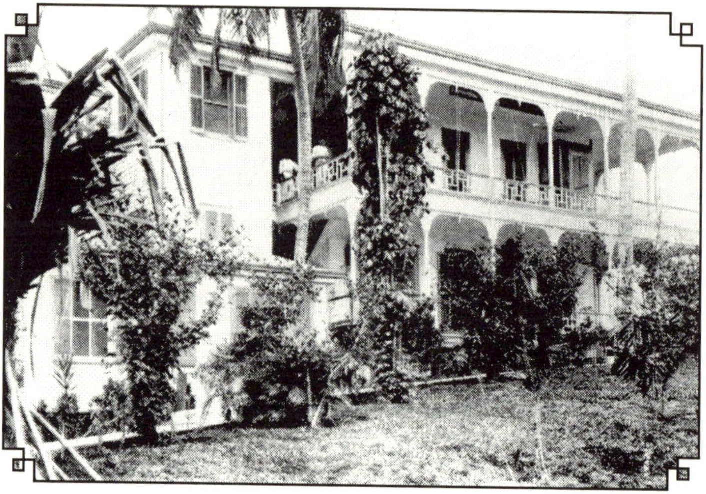

Above: East side of Main Hospital (right) and Annex.

Below: Nurse in staff quarters.

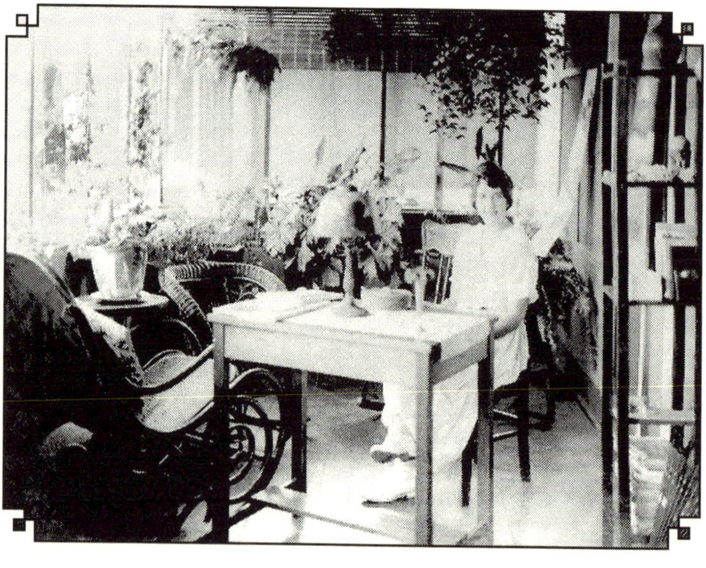

pital for laborers. After the Colored Hospital was completed, the upper floor of the Annex became a kitchen where food was prepared and served in the adjoining Main Hospital.

Residence of Manager/ Medical Superintendent

Originally, John Morgan Kyes, the Division Manager, lived with his wife in this spacious home until about 1913. Carlos Reid was their cook in 1912 and wrote about activities at Hospital Point. When Kyes moved to the new manager's home in the new mainland port of Almirante, the island home became the residence of the Medical Superintendent.

This building was built on a steep slope which dropped off into the sea. The main floor was surrounded on all four sides by a porch. On the east side, a long living room ran the full length of the house. Underneath the main floor were three servants' quarters, a bathroom and a washroom which were accessed from the south end. According to Bruce Brown, who lived in the servants quarters with his mother from 1908 to 1919, there was a recreation room for the doctors on the north side adjacent to the servants quarters.[19] After work, doctors would enter this game room from the lower sidewalk on the north end. They played pool, smoked cigars and had a few drinks. Meals were served to the doctors on the south-

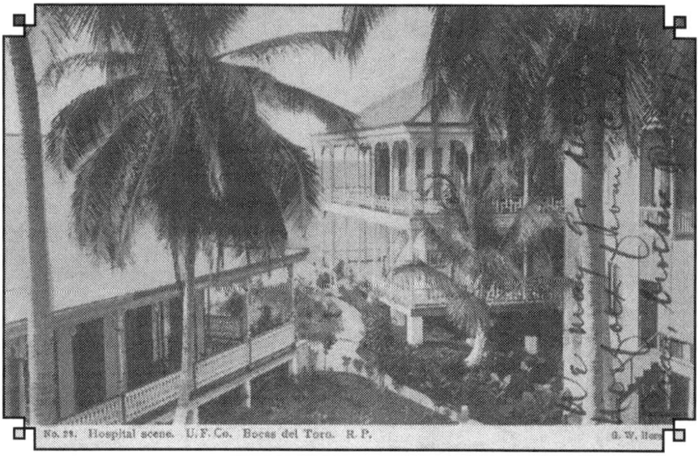

Above: Manager's residence, later home of the Medical Superintendent (left), Main Hospital (center), and Annex (right). Photograph taken from the Colored Hospital looking north.

Top right: Living room of Manager's / Doctor's House, running entire length of east side.

Below: Looking south from Hospital Point. Former Manager's House (right) later became the Medical Superintendent's House. Colored Hospital (center, rear).

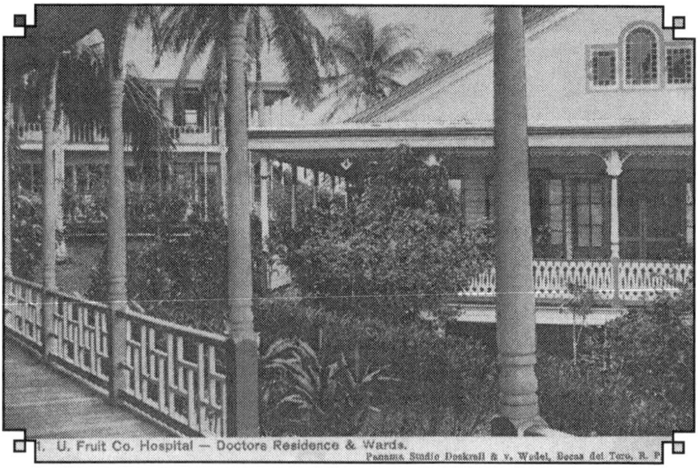

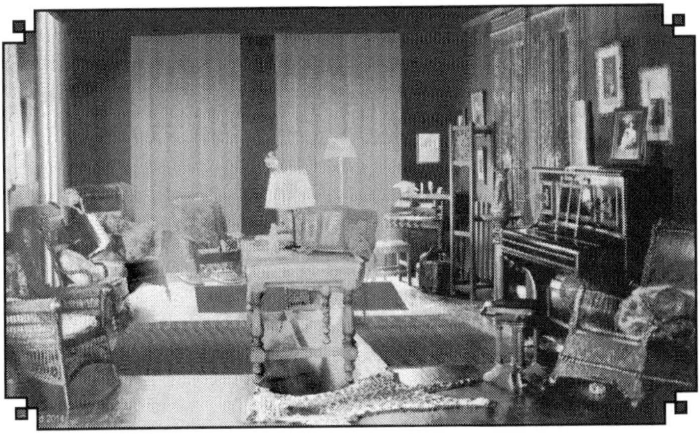

west veranda of the main floor which extended out over the rocky cliff. If the weather was bad, the shutters on the veranda were closed. There was also a dining room inside.

Kitchen

A covered walkway connected the kitchen to the Medical Superintendent's house where the food was served.

Colored Hospital

This two-story building was constructed on the highest hill (8.8 meters above sea level) and treated the labor class. The structure was known as the Colored Hospital because a majority of the work force was imported from the West Indies, mostly from Jamaica. Ward 1 was located on the second floor where tuberculosis patients were treated. A medical supply room occupied the southwest corner upstairs and was open underneath. Ward 2, known as the *Fever Ward,* was located on the first floor where malaria cases were isolated. Before 1914, the operating room and office were also downstairs on the west side. On the east side, there were two private rooms for higher class outsiders.

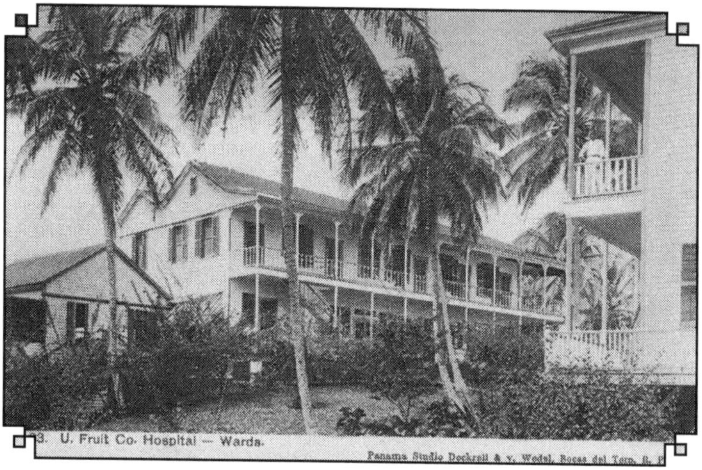

Colored Hospital (center), Warehouse (left), Annex (right).

Dining Room and Kitchen

This building had four doors on the north side for the entrance of patients. No patients were served in bed if they could walk to the dining room. Another door was located on the southwest corner to enter a separate dining room for laborers. A bakery was located on the east end of the building. Two large stoves, each with a tall chimney, originally burned coal but later used local mangrove charcoal.

Wards 3 and 4

This building was located southwest of the Colored Hospital. Ward 3 was a large open room on the second floor and was for middle and higher class non-company patients. The entrance was by the stairs on the outside of the northeast corner. This ward was not used much. Ward 4 on the first floor was for post-surgery recovery of all classes of patients. The single room was open except for privacy partitions between beds. Convalescence after surgery was enjoyed on the open air concrete floor at the north entrance which was sheltered overhead by Ward 3. Two large water tanks on the south side stored rain water collected from the roof.

Cottage

This cottage was perched on a steep slope behind Wards 3 and 4. Norman Sparks, a maintenance man, lived in the north room, and lab assistant Joseph Cox lived in the south room. Meals were served to them and certain other employees on the front porch. The bathroom was downstairs.

Laundry

Yew Lee, his brother, Sam Lee, and Chino Francisco did the laundry downstairs for the hospitals and the dining room. These three Chinese lived upstairs. Later, the laundry was contracted to residents of Old Bank on Bastimentos Island.

Laborers' House

Workers from the kitchen slept in this two-room building, also known as the *Bone House*. Dice games, played with bone dice, caused wild excitement in this house on payday. Losers would row their dugouts home to Bastimentos or Bocas completely broke. Boxing matches were also held here.

Workshop

Repairs and carpentry of all types were done here, including the building of coffins by Norman Sparks and his helpers.

Toilet

This public outhouse behind the morgue was completely over the water.

Morgue

On the east side, a viewing room was provided with a glass partition which helped to reduce the smell of dead bodies. The floor was sloped towards the southwest so body fluids from the corpses could drain into the sea.

Carbide Gas Plant

Carbide gas provided lights for Hospital Point until 1918 when the electric plant was installed.

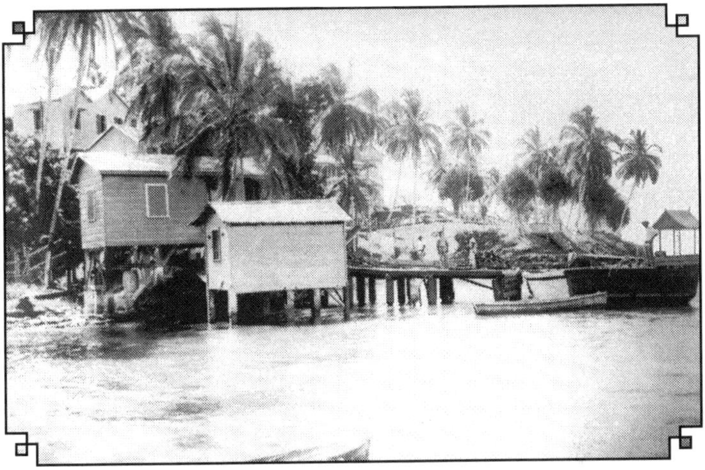

The toilet (small building over the water), the morgue (behind the toilet). The roof of the carbide plant (behind the morgue). The Main Hospital (center rear), the kitchen (upper left), the cargo dock (right of the toilet), the roof of the passenger dock (far right). Circa 1912.

Warehouse / Ice House

This building appears in earlier photographs. Materials were dispatched from a counter on the southwest corner. Later, the warehouse was removed and a large water tank was built on the north side, downhill from another water tank. The concrete ice house remained. Ice came from the plant in Bocas del Toro until a new ice plant was constructed in Almirante. When the launch delivered ice each Monday, Zachariah "Iron Man" Brown and Philip "Big Man" Manuel vied to see who could push three large blocks of ice in a wheelbarrow up the steep sidewalk without stopping. Zachariah "Slim" Wray was much smaller but he always got the ice to the top. Ice cooled vegetables, meats and other perishables and served general needs in the hospitals.

Covered Sidewalk

This roof provided protection from the rain between the Colored Hospital and the new building for surgery.

New Surgery Building

Dr. I. W. McLean noted in his 1914 *Annual Report* that the new building for surgery had been completed and was completely equipped with the latest model surgical appliances. A photograph of the building appeared in the 1917 *Annual Report*. The top floor was for surgery and was entered from the covered sidewalk from the Colored Hospital. To build the lower floor, part of the steep slope had to be excavated in order to construct Allan C. Pinto's administrative medical laboratory on the east corner. These three facilities were entered from a long porch which had stairs at both ends.

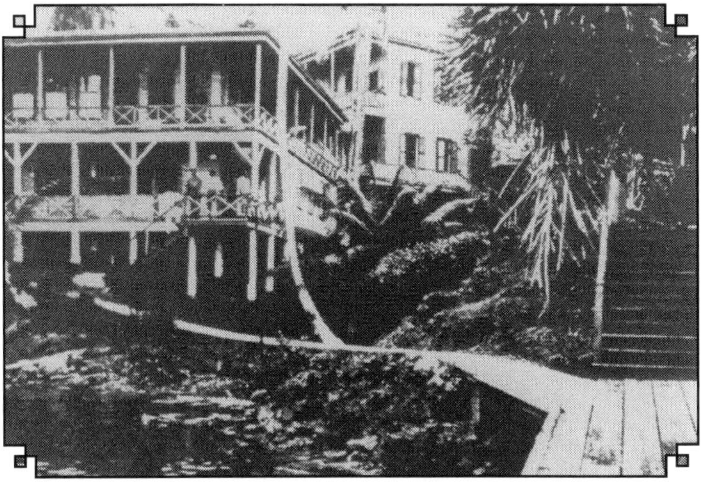

New Surgery Building, 1914. Surgery (top floor); laboratory, pharmacy, and office (first floor); Annex (center).

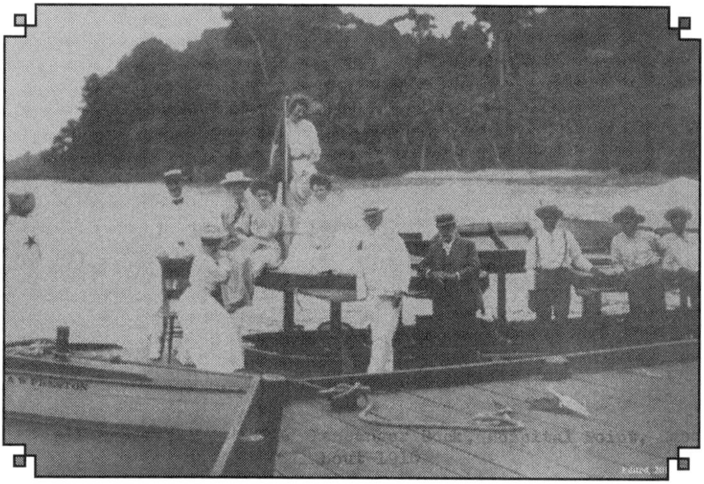

Passenger Dock, circa 1910.
Dr. I. W. McLean (left).

The Docks

Passenger Dock

Hospital Point is washed by waves from the open Caribbean and does not have a protected anchorage. Rails for concrete pilings were driven into coral rock to support a wooden dock in less than two meters of water. Passenger launches rode the swells at dockside. Photographs dated 1910 and 1912 show the dock with a roof. The company launch departed daily from Nancy's Cay to Bocas del Toro at 6:30 AM, 11:00 AM and 5:10 PM and stayed overnight in the protected waters of Bocas del Toro at the company dock. Round trips to and from the two islands were coordinated so patients and passengers could connect with launch service to and from the mainland.

Cargo Dock

Materials and supplies were unloaded from

launches and barges. Water was less than two meters deep. Anchors or a tugboat on the deep side held barges in place during unloading. Coal for firing the kitchen stoves came in a barge and was shoveled into a small rail car waiting at the end of the dock. The loaded rail car was winched by a cable through an opening in the sidewalk at a point between the morgue and carbide gas house. A wooden draw bridge built over the sidewalk opening was raised so the car could pass and dump the coal down a wooden chute for stockpiling. To operate the winch, two men cranked a spool of cable connected to a reduction gear housed in a concrete casing.

Facilities and Services

Water

Rain water from the roofs was stored in elevated tanks and used for drinking, cooking and bathing.

Sewage and Garbage

There were no septic tanks and sewage was flushed directly into the sea. A pump behind the workshop pumped salt water to storage tanks above the second floors in order to flush toilets. Salt water corrosion was severe and resulted in the installation of a fresh water system pumped by a windmill from a well located 170 meters southeast of the medical center. Although the forest was cut down to increase wind velocity, the system did not work. Consequently, the salt water system was reconnected.[20]

Kitchen garbage and other disposable materials were thrown in the sea. Numerous glass and crock bottles, medicine bottles, crockery, broken china and junk machinery became encrusted by sponge and coral formations.

Electricity

A 110-volt generator pulled by V-belts from a Morse Fairbanks gas engine was installed in 1918 by W. E. McLaren. When Hospital Point was abandoned in 1920, this plant was moved and installed by Norman Sparks at the United Fruit Company office building in the city of Bocas del Toro. It was not until 1926 when Carl Friese, a local German merchant, was contracted by the Panama government to install a power plant for the city of Bocas del Toro. Thus, Hospital Point had electricity eight years before the capital of the province.

Sanitation

The 1914 *Annual Report* outlines precautions to promote public health. Mosquito breeding habitats were drained and treated with a larvicide formulated in an insecticide mixing plant on Hospital Point. Grass and bushes were chopped. No trees were left except coconut palms and ornamentals. Rain barrels were inspected and screened. Bottles and cans were buried. The neighboring village was inspected weekly.

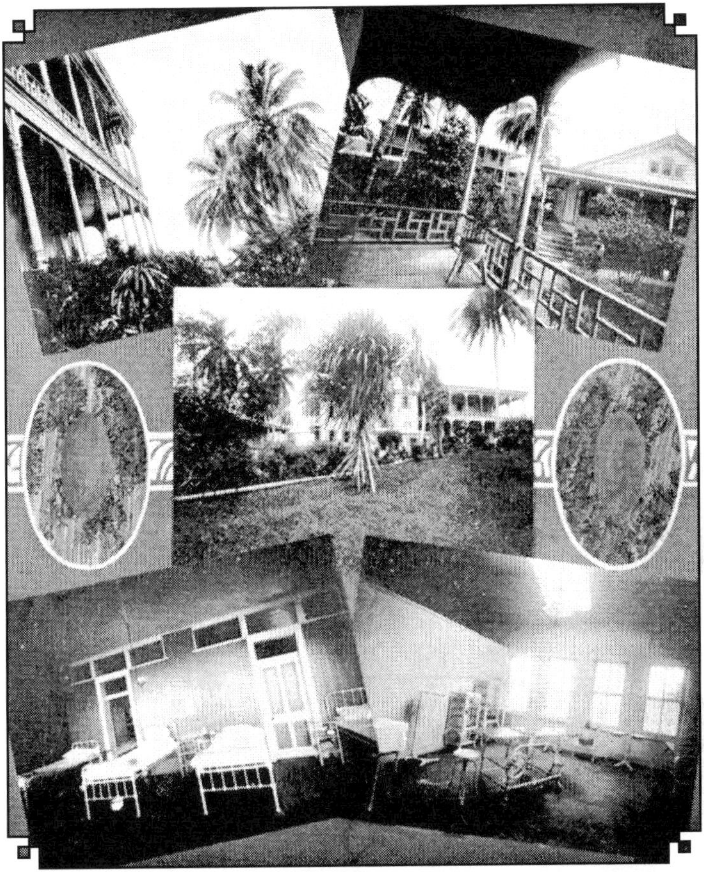

East side of Main Hospital (top left). Photograph (upper right) taken from the porch of the Main Hospital looking south at the water tank and Colored Hospital (left) and the home of the Manager / Medical Superintendent (right). Center photograph shows the east side of Main Hospital and Annex. Bottom photographs show hospital beds and clinic. Photograph from The Blue Book of Panama, 1917.

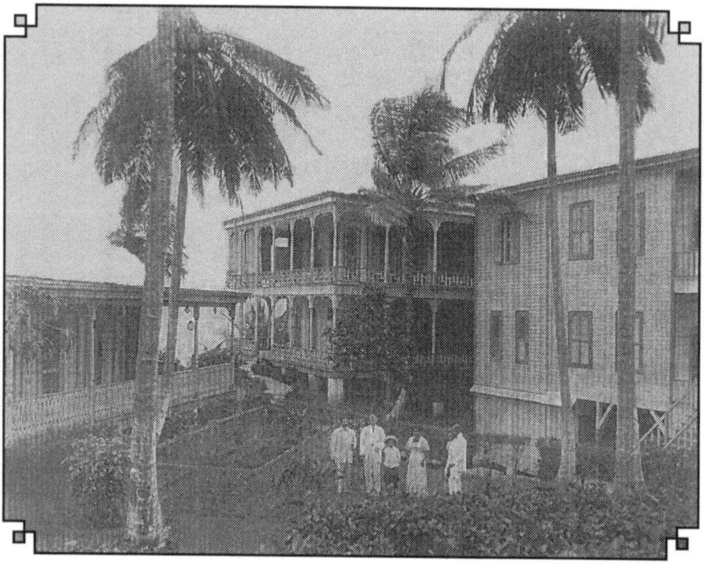

Manager John Kyes (2nd from left), his son and wife. Their house is on the left. They moved to a new house in Almirante in 1913.

Personnel

General Manager

In 1917, *The Blue Book of Panama* described the manager as follows:

> John Morgan Kyes is the manager of the Bocas del Toro Division of the United Fruit Company, an employee for 16 years. He worked previously in Costa Rica with Minor C. Keith where he advanced from the company's railroad section foreman to general roadster. He left the railroad and was promoted to assistant manager. Mr. Kyes was born in Livingston Parish, Louisiana, on January 20, 1862. He was educated in public and private schools in Louisiana and was married in 1888. The couple has two sons, Lee Charlton and Owen Stanley. Mr. Kyes is a born executive.[21]

John Kyes preferred to live on Nancy's Cay in a luxurious home and commute daily on his company launch to the United Fruit Company office in Bocas del Toro. He also made trips to review company operations on the mainland. About 1913, he moved to the new manager's home in Almirante.

Early Doctors

Two doctors died soon after Hospital Point was opened. They were buried in the German cemetery near Bocas del Toro and their tombstones read:

- Clarence G. Probert, M.D. Born August 30, 1871. Died June 28, 1901.
- John Eccles, M.D., Age 51 years, 5 months, 24 days. Born in Madras, India, July 24, 1850. Died in Bocas del Toro, Colombia, January 18, 1902.

Medical Directors

Robert Earl Swigart, the first medical director, stated:

> The struggles of this division directly after the organization of the United Fruit Company in 1899, through revolution, pestilence, wind storms and floods, mark an era in sanitary development. The sanitary procedures incident to Dr. Walter Reed's findings in Cuba were inaugurated here under the Colombian regime of Panama, and before the Americans came to build the Panama Canal in 1904.[22]

Data substantiates that Dr. Swigart was the

pioneer doctor in controlling tropical diseases in Bocas del Toro so that the United Fruit Company could develop the banana business.

According to early reports, Dr. Swigart and his wife lived in the Main Hospital. He also owned two houses on the hill northwest of the white cemetery. One house was rented and the other was occupied by an Austrian overseer of the 150-hectare Swigart farm east of Pine Creek. In the 1912 *Annual Report* (Volume 1), Swigart reviewed the history of medical problems and services in Bocas del Toro from 1899 to 1911. This report was dated September 30, 1911, in Bocas del Toro. The following year, he was promoted to General Superintendent under a new organization authorized January 1, 1912, as head of all medical activities in the company. His letter of transmittal in the same volume was dated December 1, 1912, in New Orleans and was directed to Andrew W. Preston, President of the United Fruit Company, Boston. Swigart's 1913 *Annual Report* was submitted from New York and stated that he was obliged to spend six months in the tropics reviewing medical programs for the company's 65,000 employees and dependents. It was noted that the death-rate had improved to a level the same as in more advanced countries, and that there were no quarantinable diseases that year. He reorganized medical services for the 90 company steamships.

Swigart wrote his last annual report from New York on October 1, 1914. In the 1915 *Annual Report* submitted from New York, the new General Superintendent, Dr. William E. Deeks, reported the death of Dr. Swigart. Deeks praised Swigart's pioneer work in the tropics and his organization of the Medical Department.

When Swigart left Bocas del Toro in 1912, he was replaced by Dr. I. W. McLean. The new doctor was born on November 15, 1880, in Charlotte, North Carolina. McLean studied medicine at the University of Maryland and then became a surgeon in Panama during the construction of the Panama Canal. He was a member of the Canal Zone Medical Association. The 1912 *Annual Report* lists his Hospital Point staff as follows:

- Dr. I. W. McLean, Superintendent, Baltimore Medical College
- Dr. R. H. Wilson, Assistant Surgeon, Starling Medical College
- Dr. J. E. Smith, Pathologist, Tulane University
- Dr. C. S. Carter, District Medical Officer, University of Tennessee
- C. B. Lawrence, Matron

Table 1 lists 70 other employees as shown in the 1913 *Annual Report*. The report also showed that the Medical Department was responsible for providing health care for the following: white employees, 300; families of white employees, 200; black employees, 6,000; families of black employees, 5,000.

Table 1. Positions of 70 employees of the Medical Department in 1913

Matron, Main Hospital	1	Attendants	16
Chief Nurse, Colored Hospital	1	Maids	2
Assistant Chief Nurse, Colored Hospital	1	Mechanic	1
Druggist	1	Carpenters	2
Dispensers	5	Painter	1
Laboratory Assistant	1	Linen Keeper	1
Storekeeper	1	Waiter	1
Assistant Storekeeper	1	Laborers	2
Storeman	1	Yardmen	5
Medical Nurses	7	Launderers	5
Surgical Nurses	2	Bakers	2
Cooks	7	Launchmen	3

McLean had been a bachelor until he brought back a young wife after a vacation. They soon had a baby at Hospital Point. According to Bruce Brown, he was a reserve officer who reported to duty during World War I. His packing boxes were addressed as Captain I. W. McLean. In 1918, Dr. Deeks confirmed that 10 doctors of the United Fruit Company had been commissioned in the military service to serve in the war. Three of these were medical superintendents that had resigned that year. After the war, McLean was appointed as Medical Superintendent for the United Fruit Company at Port Antonio, Jamaica, on May 1, 1919.

Dr. C. F. Watson, of Vanderbilt University, replaced McLean in 1918. His publication in the *Annals of Surgery* reported the first case in Panama of trematodes in the gall bladder of a Chinaman. The parasite is a liver fluke common in China and Japan. He also published on "Intestinal obstruction due to *Ascaris lumbricoides*" and "Gauze sponge in abdomen for 14 years; Ectopic gestation simulated." Dr. Watson was in charge when Hospital Point was closed and the new hospital in Almirante opened on September 1, 1920.

Other Staff Members

While most of the doctors and head nurses were Americans, many of the supporting staff were well-trained Jamaicans educated in British colonial schools. Others, like Jamaican employee, Alan C. Pinto, climbed the ladder of success on their own. Originally, Pinto was a water boy on a local banana boat. When he spent a long time at the hospital recovering from an injury, he impressed the right people. The young man went to school and studied special courses. Eventually, he became the chief administrator and developed a model card catalog file system.

Norman Sparks, a Jamaican, and a *Jack of all Trades*, handled most any kind of work task at Hospital Point. His helpers were two Jamaicans named Sam Joseph and "Father" Lewin.

Rebecca Francis Swartz, a local Creole, lived in the maid's room under the Medical Superintendent's house from 1908 to 1919. She was a servant for manager John Kyes, and later for the doctors who lived in the house. On one occasion, she accompanied the Herbert Leer family to Germany as a nanny. (Leer was a United Fruit Company official and prominent German merchant in Bocas del Toro.) Rebecca Swartz was born on the neighboring island of Bastimentos in 1879. Her father was Robert Swartz, born on Corn Island, Nicaragua, and her mother was Maggie Machore from British Honduras. In 1906, Rebecca Swartz had a son, Bruce Brown. His father, whose name was Brown, was an English steward on a ship that loaded bananas in Bocas del Toro, but the boy never knew his father. (This version was written on Bruce Brown's baptismal record. However, he learned from his family that his real father was Egers Dorffer, a German from Hamburg. Dorffer worked in Herbert Leer's store. Herbert Leer and his wife took Rebecca Swartz with them on a German ship from Bocas del Toro to Germany as a nanny for their two children. Egers Dorffer was also on that voyage. Thus, Bruce was a Dorffer, not a Brown.) It was Bruce's step-father, Norman Sparks, who helped to raise and motivate the boy.

Hospital Point was a playground for Bruce Brown and he knew everybody and everything that was going on at the medical center. As a young child, Bruce wore long hair and was dressed in a long smock. After his hair was finally cut, Mrs. Swigart remarked with a hilarious laugh, "I always thought you were a little girl, but now I'm seeing a little boy!"

When Bruce was 11, he almost went to school in the United States. Dr. I. W. McLean was leaving for World War I and had planned to sponsor the boy in an American school. As Bruce and the doctor were boarding the company launch at Hospital Point to transfer to a banana ship sailing to the USA, the American Consul and Panama quarantine officer, Dr. Paul Osterhout, was advised of the boy's trip abroad. In a loud and stern voice, Osterhout exclaimed, "Can't be done!" There was no explanation and the disappointed boy stayed behind, never to see his benefactor again.

Bruce Brown entered school when he was 10. Many students went to Bocas del Toro to the "pay school" which was taught in English by Jamaicans educated under the British school system. However, Bruce went to the free public school even though he did not speak Spanish. He caught the daily launch at 6:00 AM and returned late in the afternoon. The teacher put him in the second grade because he was too big and too old for the first grade. When Hospital Point closed down in 1920, Bruce and his family moved to the neighboring village at Diego Point. He sailed a sawmill dugout across the channel to school in Bocas del Toro. Bruce was a fast learner and graduated from the sixth grade at the the top of his class. Eventually, he became a laboratory technician in the Almirante hospital under Dr. Otto Brosius.

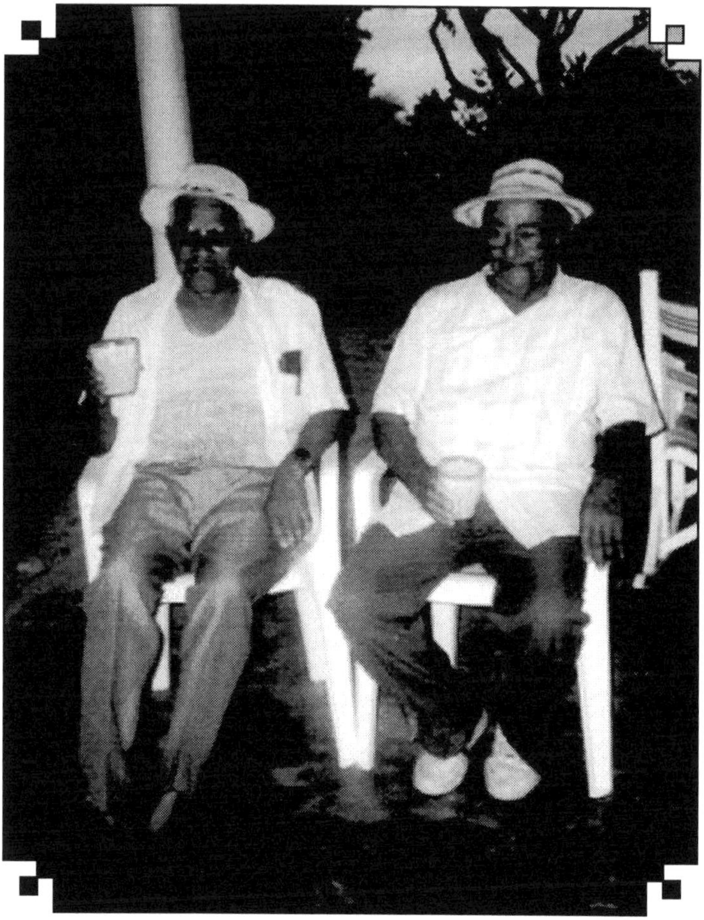

Bruce Brown (right) with his half-brother Martin Sparks (left), chatting with the author on Hospital Point, 1990s.

Recreation

ROLLING DICE, PLAYING CARDS, boxing, playing music, singing and fishing were favorite pastimes. Target shooting with a .22 caliber rifle was popular on the little point by the Chinese store and prizes were awarded to the best marksman. There was a launch to Bocas del Toro to see the movies at the Broadway Theater. On weekends, many would take the launch to Almirante and transfer to a special train to the border town of Guabito to attend the horse races at Henry Blair Park. Men dressed in black suits, white shirts and ties. Bets on the races were two dollars. Race horses were imported and trained at Farm Six in Changuinola. Horses were also raced on the beaches at Bocas del Toro.

Americans were highly competitive in the United Fruit Company baseball league but West Indians did not play baseball. Their heritage from the British was cricket. Cricket teams from Bocas del Toro, Careening Cay, Bastimentos, Hospital Point, Almirante, Changuinola and Guabito competed. There was a cricket field on Nancy's Cay at Diego Point.

A well-drained clay tennis court was built on the only flat surface of Hospital Point. Since all the trees had been cleared, the sun usually dried the court enough to play on. On one occasion, Dr. McLean invited Zachariah "Iron Man" Brown to practice with him. "Iron Man" lived up to his reputation and hit the ball far out to sea. The ball was never recovered, but the story became legendary.

Medical History

MEDICAL INFORMATION ABOUT HOSPITAL Point was recorded in several books, but statistical details were published in the United Fruit Company Medical Department annual reports. Volume 1 began in 1912 and included updated reports from 1899. The 1920 report covered the last year at Hospital Point. This series ended with Volume 20 in 1931, a period of economic depression. All 20 volumes are in the Countway Library of Medicine at Harvard University. Each volume covers reports from all medical departments in banana and sugarcane divisions scattered throughout the tropics, plus medical reports from company ships of the Great White Fleet.

Reports stated that yellow fever was rampant in the 1890s and remained endemic in Chiriquicito and Bocas del Toro until 1903. Strict control measures eliminated this disease. The last death from yellow fever was in 1906. Malaria was greatly reduced but hundreds of cases were still reported each year. For example, 1,228 cases were treated in the company hospitals in 1908-09 and another 5,557 cases were treated in the plantation dispensaries that year. In 1903, 122 cases of smallpox were isolated during an epidemic in the province. The disease was wiped out by banana company doctors who vaccinated 7,000 people. It was noted that only blacks were affected. Dr. W. E. Deeks stated that 40–100% of lowland tropical populations were debilitated with hookworms, which are sometimes fatal, and combined with malaria, produced much acute morbidity among populations. He also stressed the losses from dysentery and amoebic dysentery. Pneumonia, kidney disease, and tuberculosis were common causes of death. In his 1915 *Annual Report*, Dr. I. W. McLean listed the six principal diseases among laborers in order of importance: malaria, venereal diseases, pneumonia, nephritis, uncinariasis, and tuberculosis. He also stated that 24 incurables had been assisted to their homes in the West Indies that year.

Carlos Reid recalls that the company launch made two trips daily between Almirante, Bocas del Toro and Hospital Point, often bringing up to 10 patients from the mainland farms with snakebites and malaria, known as *blackwater fever*. In labor communities, public health was greatly improved by providing schools, churches and plots to grow home gardens. In the company churches, chaplains imported from Jamaica were expected to preach both salvation and sanitation. Schools also emphasized sanitation and good health.

During the year 1908-09, 582 white patients were admitted to the hospitals and nine died. This compared with 3,155 colored patients admitted and 91 died. A third of the colored patients admitted had malaria. That same year, 18,508 treatments of employees were recorded at the dispensaries, which included an outpatient dispensary on Hospital Point. Of all admissions that year, patients came from 55 countries, plus other miscellaneous nationalities listed for 260 patients. Of the colored patients, 2,017 were from Jamaica, 99 were from the French-speaking islands of Martinique, Guadeloupe and Haiti, and 56 came from the United States of America. The remainder of colored patients came from India, Africa, Central and South America, and many islands in the Caribbean. Of the 582 white patients, 295 were from the United States and the remaining 287 came from 36 other countries. In the operating room, 47 types of surgery were performed on 310 patients.

Deaths, Burials and Cemeteries

CARLOS REID, BRUCE BROWN and Enos Fleming referred to half a dozen deaths a day and that probably was the case on some days. However, after 1909, the highest annual death-rate recorded in the annual reports was 87 in 1920. In 1914, the death-rate increased because of the arrival of old and disabled men who had been released after the Panama Canal was completed. During that year, the principal causes of the 86 deaths were as follows: tuberculosis 7, chronic nephritis 12, acute nephritis 4, pneumonia 23, pernicious estivo-autumnal malaria 8, pernicious tertian malaria 1, cerebral estivo-autumnal malaria 2, typhoid fever 1, pellagra 2, heart disease 9, beriberi 2, external violence 4, and the other 11 from miscellaneous diseases.

Annual reports noted the deaths of Americans as follows:

- R. N. Coates, engineer, 2 years residence, age 38, hemoglobinuria fever, buried in Nancy's Cay cemetery, 1913.
- J. E. Campbell, overseer, 28 months of residence, age 26, killed by gunshot, buried in Nancy's Cay cemetery, 1913.
- B. F. Willis, overseer, 8 months of residence, age 38, thrown from a mule, 1914.

Coffins were built in the shop by Norman Sparks, "Father" Lewin and Sam Joseph. Contracts for digging the grave and making the burial were given to Sam Galero, Peter Hudson, Alfonso Ponier and Dawson, who earned five dollars per burial. Originally, a coffin was put on a two-wheeled cart and pulled by two men down the trail through Nancy's Cay Village to the colored cemetery just beyond Diego Point. However, local residents petitioned the company to change the route because of the smells and unpleasantness of dead bodies passing by their homes so frequently.

The company agreed and the cart was replaced by a flat, open, copper-bottom barge, built on a wooden frame. The boat was known as the *Dead Skiff* and it held two coffins which were loaded from the cargo dock by the morgue. A pair of oarsmen rowed the skiff around Hospital Point to Diego Point. In 1992, wave action partially uncovered this relic skiff buried 72 years beneath the sand and turtle grass south of the cargo dock. It measured eight meters long by 2.5 meters wide.

Burials in the company-owned colored cemetery were made in the clay hills above the mangrove beach beyond Diego Point. Many of the dead had families only back in their country of origin. Each grave was marked with a wooden stake with an identification number. The number referred to a file kept in the hospital office. Rot and termites destroyed the markers in less than a year. Today, there is no sign of this cemetery. Indigenous families living on and near these hills are unaware of an estimated one thousand burials under their village.

The white cemetery is on the opposite side of the island on the north shore, 175 meters southeast of the old tennis court site on a hill above the cliff near Pine Creek. This burial ground was well-kept and had a neat white picket fence around it. A wire fence marked the one-hectare boundary of the company-owned plot. Dr. Swigart's two houses on the hill and the windmill and well in the valley below were also within this property line.

After the medical center closed in 1920, the graveyard grew back into jungle. In 1993, the burial ground was cleaned and each tombstone was inventoried (Table 2). It appears that some burials never had permanent markers. Several graves have elaborate marble or granite tombstones but others have concrete and gravel stones which were molded locally. These were marked with a metal plate embedded in the concrete.

The earliest marked grave is dated 1908 and the last was August 22, 1920, just before the hospital closed. Data of several of the deceased has been recorded. Emile Moses was a paymaster in Bocas and also sold tickets for the company launch. In 1913, R. N. Coates, engineer, age 38, American, two years of residence, died from hemoglobinuric fever. J. E. Campbell, a farm overseer, died from gunshot wounds. T. A. Timlin was a railroad man from Pennsylvania and was chief storekeeper of materials and supplies when he died at age 31.

Three isolated graves, 20 meters to the southwest, were found in the jungle. In 1917, Effie Louise Roberts and Audrey Coul White died as a result of a serious railcar accident near the Sixaola River railroad bridge which crossed from Panama to Costa Rica. Both women were buried side by side. Based on a biographical sketch in *The Blue Book of Panama*, Mrs. Roberts and her husband, Neill S. Roberts, lived in a huge plantation house isolated on the hill above Margarita Farm on the Costa Rican side of the Sixaola River. He was born in Tennessee in 1880, became a timekeeper in 1901, and was superintendent of farms. The couple married in 1912 and had one son.

R. E. White, husband of the other deceased woman, was born in Iowa in 1862, graduated from

Brown University, and married Audrey Coul in Rhode Island in 1887. He advanced from timekeeper to General Superintendent of the Guabito farms. The couple lived in a spacious house in Guabito. After her death, White came on weekends to weep upon her grave and talk to her. His grief was observed by Bruce Brown from the Swigart farm house by the cemetery. When White left the country, the body was exhumed and the metal marker was taken from the concrete tombstone. Today, only broken pieces of concrete remain at the grave site.

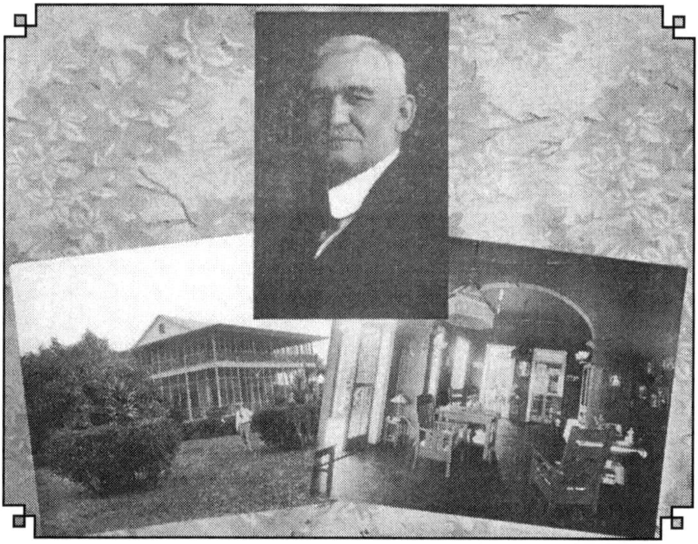

R. E. White, whose wife was buried on Nancy's Cay, and their house in Guabito.
Photographs from The Blue Book of Panama, 1917.

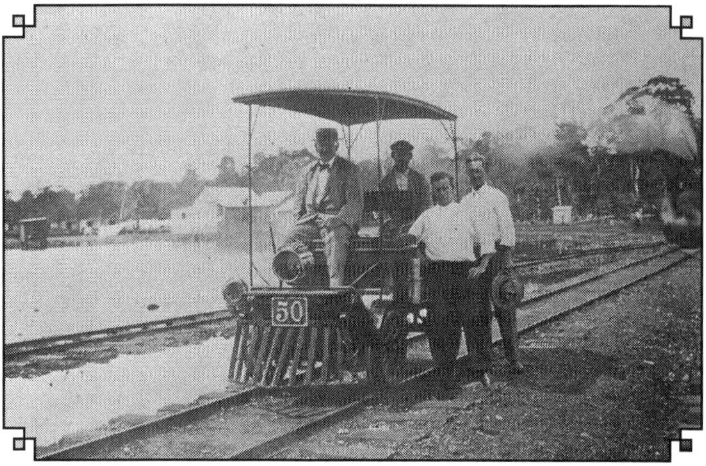

Above: Railroad Superintendent E. D. Nash (left) in Almirante, building the rail line to Changuinola.

Below: E. D. Nash's home in Empalme in Changuinola. Mr. Nash died in 1911. He was replaced by R. E. White, whose wife died in a railcar accident in 1917. She was buried near Mr. Nash in the hospital cemetery.

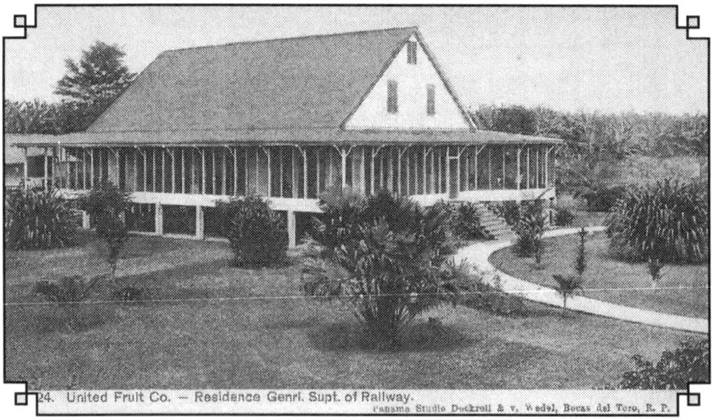

Table 2. Tombstones in the white cemetery, 1993, Nancy's Cay

Row 1 (West side of cemetery, graves north to south)	Infant son of J. W. and Dora Heim, Died Sunday, Aug. 22, 1920
	T. A. Timlin, Died Oct. 13, 1916
	Emile Moses, Died Jan. 17, 1917
Row 2	R. N. Coates, Died May 10, 1913
	K. A. Davidson, Died June 27, 1912
	E. D. Sundstrom, Died July 24, 1912
	C. B. Parmell, Died Oct. 14, 1909
Row 3	Infant daughter of Mr. and Mrs. C. M. Lowing, April 5-April 7, 1912
	J. Donnely, Died June 30, 1911
	L. W. Locks, Died Aug. 21, 1908
Row 4 (East side of cemetery)	Sacred to the Memory of Charles Sheridan Moseley, Born at Port Antonio, Aug. 21, 1883, Died at Bocas del Toro, April 2, 1912, R.I.P.
	J. E. Campbell, Died Dec. 9, 1913
	Lamar C., son of S. R. & Sallie Willis, Born in Cuba, Ala., Nov. 5, 1886, Died Aug. 8, 1915, Brother
Other burials in Rows 1 to 4 are not marked.	
	E. D. Nash, Died Nov. 11, 1911
	Exhumed grave of Audrey Coul White, Died 1917 (Metal plate marker removed)
	Mrs. Effie Louise Roberts, Died Jan. 15, 1917

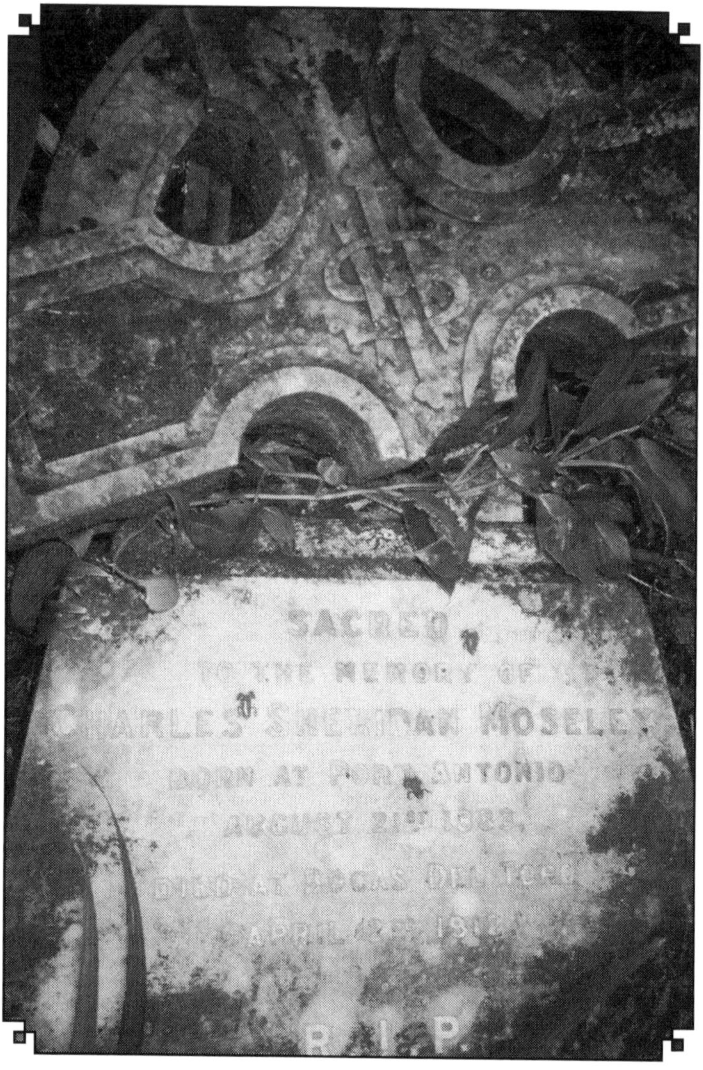

Tombstone of Charles Sheridan Moseley at Hospital Point, fallen into disrepair. Note the tiny red poison-dart frogs.

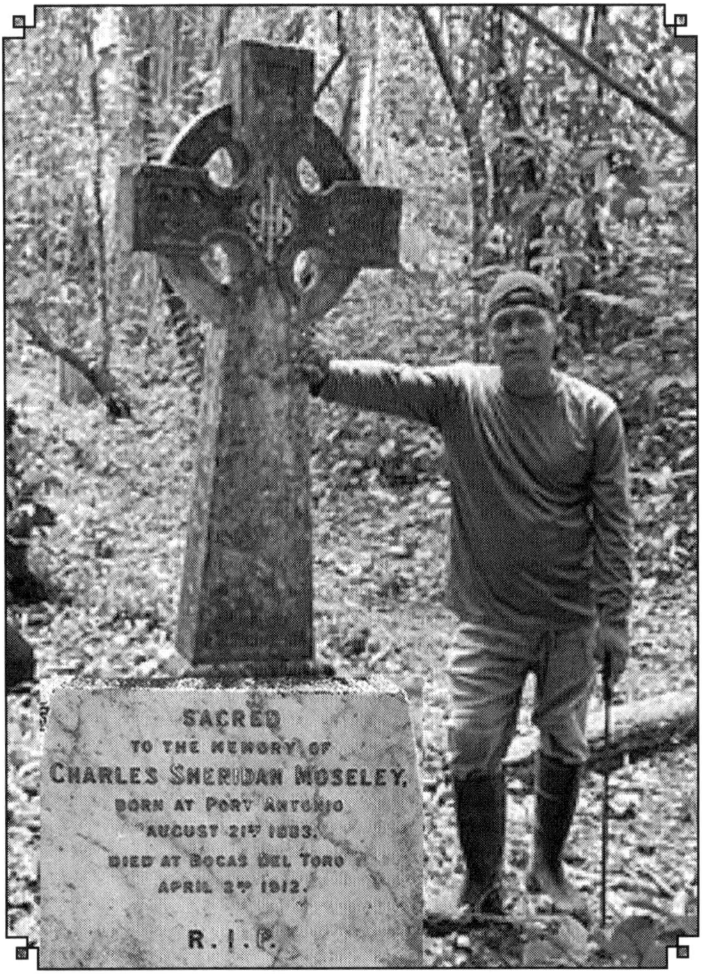

Gallic tombstone with the Gallic Cross that fell to the ground and broke into pieces because of tree damage. Years later, Leovigildo Julian Lorenzo restored the mangled tombstone almost to perfection; a remarkable feat for an indigenous person who never went to school. His father was a member of the Mama Chi cult that forbid public education of children. The author of this book and his wife Phyllis taught Leo the basics in education. He has more than proven himself in many ways over the years.

Nancy's Cay Village

A FEW CREOLE FAMILIES lived along the west shore between Hospital Point and Diego Point before the medical center was constructed. As Hospital Point developed, new residents arrived. Dr. McLean noted in the 1912 *Annual Report* that his department had control of sanitation matters in the village of 300. In a photograph taken in 1913, two dozen houses were visible along the shore.

This was an English-speaking community and most residents refused to learn or speak Spanish, which they called *that parrot language*. This attitude was demonstrated when a young woman in the village went away to improve her Spanish so she could return to teach the language in the community's Methodist church. Due to a lack of interest, her language school was a failure and closed.

Nancy's Cay people were a mixture of Caribbean cultures from Corn Island (Nicaragua), the islands of San Andres and Providencia (Colombia), British Honduras, and later, Jamaica. Beginning at Hospital Point and continuing to Diego Point, the following families were residents during the time of the hospitals, as remembered by Bruce Brown and his wife, Lillian Campbell de Brown. Most of these people were native-born Creoles of African descent:

> Peter Hudson, Octavia Hudson La Cruz, James Kennedy, Marionette Hudson de Roderick Smith, Isadora Hudson de Correa; all brothers and sisters and children of Fidelia Hudson, from British Honduras, who was the community mid-wife; Mrs. Correa, Miss Foster, Mr. Dawkins, James Dixon, Fanny Sammuels, and Melina Bryan.

Land was communally owned but home plots were passed on to relatives without legal papers or problems. Most residents were Methodist. The Reverend M. C. Surgeon, a Jamaican, came from Bocas del Toro to preach. He stayed in the overnight house which was owned by Isadora Hudson de Correa and was located south of the tennis court. Carlos Reid also preached in the church on the hill 200 meters south of Hospital Point. Crime was unheard of, people were honest, and nobody locked their doors.

There were two Chinese stores built over the

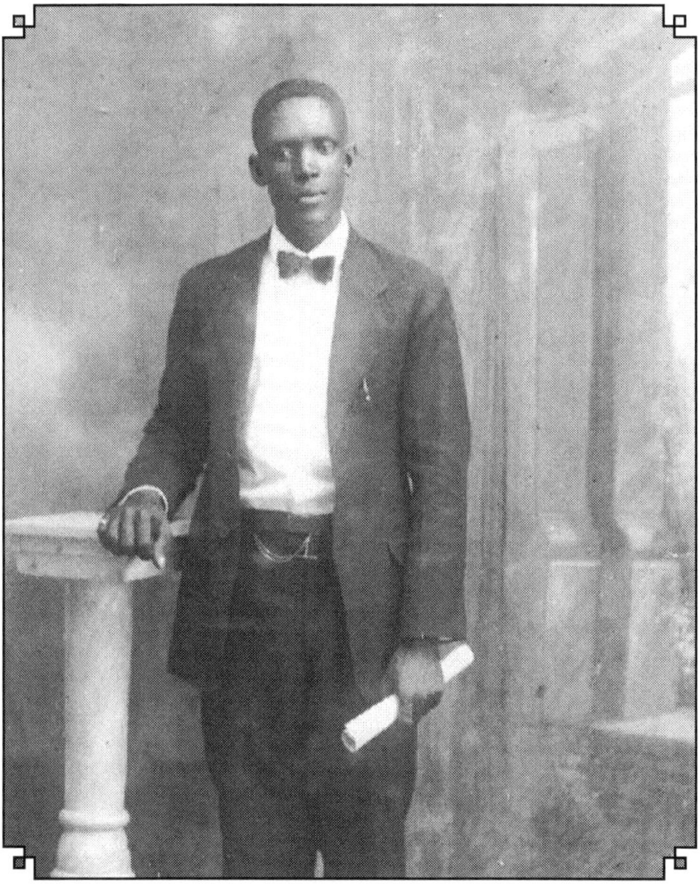

Carlos Reid, age 35, 1928

water on the west shore adjacent to Hospital Point. No one knew the real name of one shopkeeper but everybody called him Chino Peyne. This name came from the fact that the man walked with a painful limp, thus the name "pain eh!" He lived with a local woman in their store. This store sold general merchandise but no alcohol. It was also a gathering place for the locals. Charles Adams, a lab assistant in the hospital, had an argument with the gravedigger, Alfonso Ponier. Adams shot Ponier through the shoulder but the bullet went on and hit Chino Peyne in his store, causing him even more pain. Adams was put in the Bastimentos jail for a short time.

The other Chinese shop and home was about 30 meters south of Chino Peyne's store. This business was owned by James Tong, a more refined English type. He later moved his store to Pumpkin River.

Peter Hudson was the lawman on the island but had nothing to do. People respected each other and there was no stealing. However, young Bruce Brown, who was always playing like a sailor at the docks, released the lines of the company launch too quickly one day and caused some aggravation. Peter Hudson put Bruce in jail to teach him a lesson. Jail was nothing more than an empty room in a house. Bruce soon escaped and Mr. Hudson dropped the case.

Adjacent to the community was Dr. Swigart's farm. After the doctor died in 1915, the 150-hectare farm was sold to Elmer Deems, Sr., the father of Elmer Deems, Jr., a United Fruit Company employee. Their Tropical Plantation Company produced fruits, vegetables, meat and milk for the Bocas market. A fine home was built at the top of the highest cliff on the north coast and was reached by climbing vertical stairs from the boat landing. The Deems family left in the 1920s, and the farm grew back into jungle. Eduardo Thomas acquired this land in the 1960s by paying its back-taxes. In 1973, it was sold to William Bizich. Today, there are several dozen indigenous families and a school at Diego Point.

Epilogue

THE AUTHOR AND HIS WIFE, Phyllis, bought Hospital Point from Eduardo Thomas in 1970 and retired there in 1991. Their retirement home has solar power, rain water and the first septic tank ever built on the island.

Acknowledgments

I THANK THOMAS J. Bendiburg Snyder for showing me Hospital Point from a dugout in 1966. In 1970, *don* Cipriano Castillo kindly helped me to excavate the Hospital Point ruins buried in the jungle for 50 years. I am grateful to Bruce Brown of Bocas del Toro, who provided numerous personal details about Hospital Point, and to his wife, Lillian Campbell de Brown, who related information about old families in the village. Bonnie Fay Johnson, librarian in Indianapolis, Indiana, helped begin the search for references. Lynn Badger, librarian at the University of Florida, Gainesville, and Dr. Elizabeth Swain, of Harvard University, were indispensable in obtaining old United Fruit Company medical records from the Harvard library. Virgilio Pineda and Victor Ibarra contributed to the survey and map. Larry Mahan, of Marstons Mills, Massachusetts, generously provided photographs. Professional advice from Drs. Carlos Fitzgerald, Robert H. Fusion, Samuel Gutierrez, Stanley Heckadon-Moreno and Eugene Lyon was appreciated. As usual, Silvia Chong Howard, of Bocas del Toro, devoted long hours of her personal time with the translation to Spanish. Angel and Michelle Gonzales, Antonio Manzanares, Carol Wilson, Walter Hamer, Sue Trafton Hamer, my wife, Phyllis, and our children, Linda and Carl, were helpful with the manuscript. To all of these people, I am very grateful.

References

1. Morison, Samuel E. *Admiral of the Ocean Sea*. Boston: Little, Brown and Co., 1942.
2. Fusion, Robert H. Temple Terrace, FL, USA. Personal communication, 1995.
3. Colón, Hernando. *Historia de Almirante*, Edición de Luis Arranz. Madrid: Rancor, S.A., 1984.
4. Rumeu de Armas, Antonio. *Libro copiador de Cristóbal Colón*. Madrid: Testimonio Compañía Editorial, 1987.
5. Roberts, Orlando W. *Voyages and Excursions on the East Coast and in the Interior of Central America*. 1827. Reprinted in Gainesville: University of Florida Press, 1965.
6. United Fruit Company Medical Department Annual Reports. Vols. 1-9, 1912-20.
7. Reverte, José M. *Los Indios Teribes de Panamá*. Panamá: La Estrella de Panamá, 1967.
8. Gutiérrez, Samuel A. *La arquitectura en dos archipiélagos caribeños*. Panamá: 1967.
9. Stephens, Clyde S. *Bosquejo histórico del cultivo del banano en la provincia de Bocas del Toro (1880-1980)*. Panamá: *Revista Panameña de Antropología*, 1987.

10. Stephens, Clyde S. *Bananeros in Central America.* Ft. Myers, Florida: Press Printing Co., 1989.
11. Adams, Frederick U. *Conquest of the Tropics.* New York: Doubleday, Page and Co., 1914.
12. Abbot, Willis J. *Panama and the Canal.* New York: Syndicated Publishing Co., 1914.
13. United Fruit Company Medical Department. *Annual Report.* Vol. 1, 1912.
14. Wilson, Charles M. *Empire in Green and Gold.* New York: Greenwood Press, 1968.
15. Mahan, Lawrence. Marstons Mills, MA, USA. Personal communication, 1987.
16. Reid, Carlos. *Memorias de un criollo bocatoreño.* Edited by Stanley Heckadon-Moreno. Panamá: Asociación Panameña de Antropología, 1980.
17. "Una excursión a Bocas del Toro." Panamá: *La Estrella de Panamá,* April 1, 1904.
18. United Fruit Company Medical Department. *Annual Report.* Vol. 9, 1920.
19. Interviews at Hospital Point with Bruce Brown, 1991-95.
20. Interviews at Hospital Point with Enos Fleming, 1970-75.
21. Scoullar, William T. *The Blue Book of Panama.* The Latin American Publicity Bureau, Inc., 1916-17.
22. Crowther, Samuel. *The Romance and Rise of the American Tropics.* New York: Doubleday, Doran & Col, 1929.

The Author

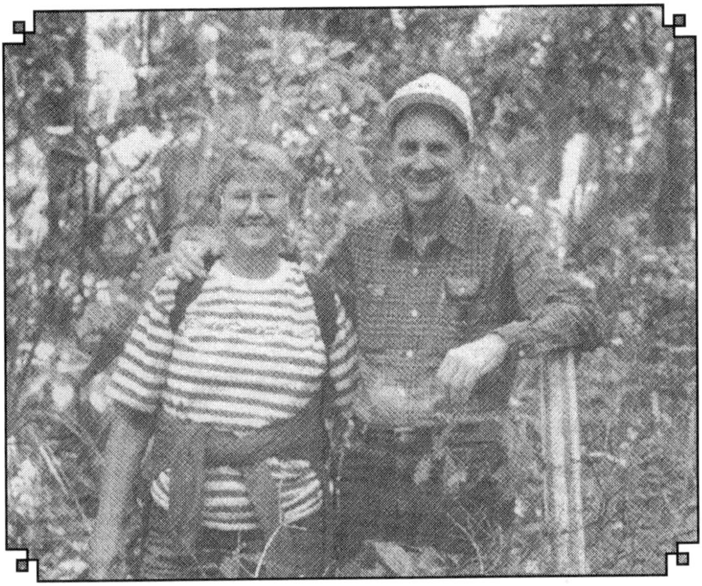

Phyllis and Clyde Stephens
Photograph by James Morris Stephens

Clyde S. Stephens, an American entomologist from Florida, USA, worked 32 years for the United Fruit Company, now Chiquita Brands International, in banana research in Central America. He has done extensive research on the history of the banana industry and has written several books on the subject. In 1991, Clyde and his wife, Phyllis, retired on Hospital Point, across the bay from where their children, Linda and Carl, were born in the banana port of Almirante, Panama.

Books by Clyde S. Stephens

Banana Man: Peeling and Revealing

Banana People

Bananeros in Central America: True Stories of the Tropics

Bosquejo histórico de la provincia de Bocas del Toro / Outline of History of the Province of Bocas del Toro, Panama

Bosquejo histórico del cultivo del banano en la provincia de Bocas del Toro (1880-1980)

La historia de Punta Hospital

History of Hospital Point

Stephens Ancestors and Pioneer Relatives

Thanks

Thank you for buying this book. I hope you enjoyed reading it as much as I enjoyed writing it. If you can, please visit wherever you bought the book and leave a review and tell your friends.

Cecropia Press
cecropiapress.com

Made in United States
Orlando, FL
14 September 2026

87741489R00053